EFFORTLESS HEALTHY EATING

Simple and Delicious Recipes for Busy Lives

Zera Schmidt

Pegmans Publishing House

CONTENTS

INTRODUCTION

Effortless Eating for Effortless Lives

Welcome to a world where delicious food and a healthy lifestyle can effortlessly coexist, even amidst the whirlwind of busy schedules! In "Effortless Healthy Eating: Simple and Delicious Recipes for Busy Lives," we embark on a journey to transform healthy eating from a daunting chore into a source of vitality, enjoyment, and well-being.

We all understand the importance of nourishing our bodies with the right foods. Countless studies published in reputable medical journals emphasise the link between a balanced diet and a multitude of health benefits. Research consistently shows that a balanced diet rich in nutrients is vital for maintaining optimal physical and mental well-being (Smith et al., 2020). A 2021 research paper published in the journal "Nutrients" also highlights the positive impact of healthy eating habits on reducing the risk of chronic diseases such as heart disease, type 2 diabetes, and even certain types of cancer (Li, Liu, Sun, Zhang, & Liu, 2021).

But let's face it, carving out time for elaborate meal prep or deciphering complicated recipes often feels like a luxury in our fast-paced lives. This book recognises that struggle. We're here to equip you with practical strategies and mouthwatering recipes that seamlessly integrate healthy eating into your busy schedule.

This isn't just another cookbook; it's your personal guide to effortless, healthy living. Whether you're a seasoned cook or a complete beginner in the kitchen, this book empowers you to make informed choices and whip up delicious, nutritious meals without sacrificing precious time.

My Personal Journey: Inspiration for Yours

My own journey towards healthy eating wasn't always smooth sailing. For years, I juggled a demanding career with the responsibilities of family life, often resorting to unhealthy convenience foods out of sheer exhaustion. The consequences, however, were undeniable: fatigue, sluggishness, and a nagging sense that I wasn't giving my body its best.

The turning point came when I discovered the power of simple, healthy meals. It wasn't about drastic changes or restrictive diets; it was about making small, sustainable adjustments. I started by incorporating more fruits and vegetables into my daily routine, a change supported by a 2020 blog post from Harvard Health Publishing that emphasises the importance of a diet rich in plant-based foods for overall health (Harvard Health Publishing, 2020). I explored quick and easy recipes that were not only delicious but also packed with nutrients. Gradually, I felt a surge of energy, improved focus, and a newfound sense of well-being.

This book is the culmination of that transformative journey. It's a collection of the knowledge I've gained, the strategies I've developed, and the delicious recipes that have fueled my own healthy lifestyle. It's also an invitation for you to embark on your own path to effortless, healthy eating.

Throughout this book, we'll delve into the fundamentals of building balanced meals, explore time-saving meal prep techniques, and discover a treasure trove of recipes tailored for busy mornings, satisfying lunches, wholesome dinners, and guilt-free treats. We'll navigate the world of healthy eating on a budget, explore sustainable food choices, and equip you with the knowledge to make informed decisions when dining out.

So, are you ready to ditch the processed foods and embrace a world of effortless, delicious, healthy eating? Let's get started!

EFFORTLESS HEALTHY EATING

Simple and Delicious Recipes for Busy Lives

CHAPTER 1

Mastering the Foundations of Healthy

Eating

Building Your Body's Powerhouse: Essential Nutrients

Let's embark on the first step towards effortless healthy eating: understanding the building blocks of a balanced diet: macronutrients and micronutrients. These powerhouses fuel our bodies, keep our minds sharp, and contribute to our overall well-being.

Macronutrients: The Power Trio

Understanding the importance of essential nutrients is the first step towards a healthier lifestyle.

first step towards a healthier lifestyle.

Carbohydrates: Often demonised but essential for energy, carbs come in two main forms: simple and complex. Simple carbs, found in sugary drinks, pastries, and white bread, provide a quick burst of energy that can lead to crashes later. Complex carbs, on the other hand, are the superstars of sustained energy. Packed with fibre, they keep you feeling fuller for longer and contribute to your digestive health. Look for complex carbs in whole grains (brown rice, quinoa), legumes (beans, lentils), fruits (apples, berries), and starchy vegetables (potatoes, sweet potatoes).

Protein is one of the building blocks of life; it is crucial for muscle growth and repair, hormone production, and a healthy immune system. A variety of protein sources ensures a balanced intake of essential amino acids. Lean protein options include chicken breast, fish (salmon, tuna), tofu, tempeh, eggs, and low-fat dairy products.

Fats: Don't let the word "fat" scare you! Healthy fats are vital for hormone regulation, brain function, and nutrient absorption. Focus on incorporating unsaturated fats like those found in avocados, olive oil, nuts (almonds, walnuts), and fatty fish (salmon, sardines). Limit saturated fats from processed meats and full-fat dairy products.

Micronutrients: The Mighty Minis

While macronutrients provide the bulk of our energy, micronutrients, including vitamins and minerals, play a crucial role in keeping our bodies functioning optimally. Additionally, it's crucial to ensure an adequate intake of essential vitamins and minerals, which play key roles in maintaining overall health and preventing deficiencies. Here are some key players:

Vitamin A supports vision, immune function, and cell growth. Found in carrots, sweet potatoes, spinach, and kale.

Vitamin C is essential for immune function, collagen production, and wound healing. Abundant in citrus fruits, bell peppers, broccoli, and strawberries.

Vitamin D aids calcium absorption for strong bones and supports immune function. Sources include fatty fish, egg yolks, and fortified foods like milk and cereals. (Sunlight exposure also contributes to vitamin D production.).

Calcium builds strong bones and teeth and supports muscle function. Found in dairy products, leafy greens (kale, collard greens), and fortified plant-based milks.

Iron carries oxygen throughout the body and is vital for energy production. Rich sources include lean red meat, poultry, fish, beans, lentils, and fortified cereals.

Building Balanced Plates: The Art Of Portion Control

Crafting well-balanced meals is essential for meeting your nutritional needs and promoting overall health. Aim to include a variety of nutrient-dense foods from all food groups in each meal. Fill your plate with colourful fruits and vegetables, lean proteins, whole grains, and healthy fats. Pay attention to portion sizes to avoid overeating, using visual cues like the size of your palm or a deck of cards to gauge appropriate serving sizes.

Now that you're familiar with the essential nutrients, let's explore how to create balanced meals using the "MyPlate" method. The MyPlate method is a simple and effective way to ensure you're incorporating a variety of essential nutrients into your meals. It is a method recommended by the USDA's ChooseMyPlate website. Imagine your plate divided into sections:

Half: Filled with non-starchy vegetables like broccoli, spinach, peppers, and leafy greens.

One-quarter: Packed with lean protein sources like grilled chicken, fish, or tofu.

One-quarter: Dedicated to whole grains like brown rice, quinoa, or whole-wheat bread.

Portion control is key to healthy eating. A helpful strategy is to visualise serving sizes. For example, a serving of protein should be about the size of your palm, while a serving of carbohydrates can be roughly the size of your fist.

Remember, this is a visual guide, not a strict rule. Customise it based on your individual needs and preferences. For example, if you're an athlete with higher protein requirements, you might adjust the protein section to be slightly larger.

Decoding The Label: Your Guide To Smart Food Choices

The grocery aisle can be a minefield, but with the right knowledge, you can navigate it with confidence. Here are some tips for deciphering food labels:

Serving Size: This is the key! Pay close attention to the serving size listed and compare it to the amount you plan to consume.

Calories: While not the sole indicator, calories provide a general idea of the energy a particular food provides.

Nutrients: Focus on the "daily value" (DV) percentages. Look for foods high in essential vitamins and minerals and low in saturated and trans fats, sodium, and added sugars.

Making Informed Choices: Putting It All Together

Armed with this knowledge, you can make informed choices at the grocery store and beyond. Here are some additional tips:

Shop the perimeter: This is where you'll find fresh produce, lean proteins, and healthy fats.

Read ingredient lists: Choose products with recognisable, whole ingredients, and limit those with a long list of processed additives.

Plan your meals: Reduce impulsive, unhealthy choices by planning your meals and creating a grocery list beforehand.

By understanding the building blocks of healthy eating, mastering portion control, and deciphering food labels, you'll be well on your way to making informed food choices. By making smart decisions and avoiding foods high in sugar, unhealthy fats, and additives, you can improve your overall health.

Quiz

A little quiz is just for you to test your knowledge and see how much you've learned about making healthier food choices.

What are your current perceptions of carbohydrates, proteins, and fats?

How do you plan to adjust your intake based on the insights shared in this chapter?

Have you ever struggled with portion control?

Write down your experiences and any strategies you've found helpful.

Take a look at the nutrition labels of three items in your pantry or fridge.

What did you learn about their nutritional content, and how might this influence your future purchasing decisions?

CHAPTER 2

Streamlining Meal Prep for Busy Lives:

Conquer your week with delicious

planning.

We all know the struggle—a busy week stretches before you, and the thought of whipping up healthy meals every night feels daunting. Fear not! Meal prep is your secret weapon for effortless, healthy eating. In this chapter, we'll unveil the time- and money-saving benefits of planning your meals, equip you with smart strategies for efficient prepping, and explore diverse meal plans for various dietary needs.

The Power Of Planning: Save Time, Save Money, And Eat Healthy

Meal planning isn't just a fad; it's a practical strategy with numerous benefits. A 2018 study published in the Journal of the Academy of Nutrition and Dietetics found that meal planning led to increased fruit and vegetable intake, reduced consumption of sugary drinks, and overall healthier food choices (Glanz et al., 2018). Here's why meal planning is your key to effortless, healthy eating:

Save Time: No more scrambling every night, wondering what to cook. Dedicate a couple of hours on the weekend to plan and prep your meals for the week, freeing up precious time during busy week-nights.

Save Money: Impulse grocery shopping often leads to wasted food and unnecessary expenses. Meal planning allows you to create a targeted grocery list, reducing food waste and saving you money.

Eat Healthier: When you have healthy meals readily available, you're less likely to resort to unhealthy convenience options during busy times.

Meal Prep Magic: Strategies For Effortless Success

Now that you're convinced of the power of planning, let's dive into the practical aspects of meal prep. Here are some key strategies for efficient and successful preparation:

Choose Your Prep Day: Dedicate a specific day (like Sunday) to meal prep. This dedicated time allows you to focus on planning, chopping, cooking, and portioning your meals for the week.

Batch cooking is your friend. Double or triple recipes to create multiple meals at once. This is a fantastic time-saving technique, especially for dishes like soups, stews, and stir-fries. Leftovers can be portioned and stored for lunches or quick dinners throughout the week.

Invest in Reusable Containers: Opt for high-quality, reusable containers to store your prepped meals. Glass containers are ideal for portion control and reheating without harmful chemicals leaching into your food.

Prioritise Freshness: Focus on prepping meals with ingredients that hold up well throughout the week. Vegetables like broccoli, carrots, and bell peppers maintain their freshness better than leafy greens, which might wilt. Store leafy greens separately and add them to meals closer to consumption.

Meal Plans For Every Lifestyle: Diversity On Your Plate

Meal planning isn't a one-size-fits-all approach. Here are some sample meal plans catering to different dietary needs:

Plant-Based Powerhouse: Focus on whole grains, legumes, vegetables, and healthy fats. This plan could include breakfast bowls with chia seeds, berries, and plant-based milk; lentil soup for lunch with a side salad; and tofu stir-fry with brown rice for dinner.

Gluten-Free Goodness: Opt for naturally gluten-free ingredients like quinoa, rice, beans, and lean proteins. Explore breakfast options like gluten-free oatmeal with fruit and nuts; lunch salads with grilled chicken or fish and quinoa; and dinners featuring baked salmon with roasted vegetables and brown rice.

Remember, these are just starting points! Customise your meal plans to fit your preferences, dietary restrictions, and readily available ingredients. Explore online resources and cookbooks for endless recipe inspiration.

With a little planning and these helpful tips, meal prep can become your secret weapon for conquering busy weeks and fuelling your body with delicious, healthy meals.

Quiz

A little quiz is just for you. Take the quiz to test your meal prep knowledge and see how you can improve your skills even further.

What obstacles do you face when it comes to meal planning?

How do you plan to overcome them after reading this chapter?

Write your favourite meal prep hack or time-saving tip.

Pick one of the sample meal plans provided and brainstorm ways to customise it to better suit your dietary preferences and lifestyle.

CHAPTER 3

Conquer Your Mornings with Energising

Breakfasts

The age-old adage "breakfast is the most important meal of the day" holds true. Starting your day with a nutritious breakfast provides a surge of energy, improves focus, and helps regulate blood sugar levels throughout the morning (Johnston, Shah, & Cassidy, 2020). But let's face it, mornings can be chaotic, leaving little time for elaborate breakfast preparations. Fear not, busy bees! This chapter is brimming with rapid and delicious breakfast inspirations designed to fuel your mornings without sacrificing precious time.

Breakfast On The Go: Quick And Nutritious Options

Here are some fantastic breakfast ideas that can be whipped up in minutes, perfect for those mornings when time is tight:

Greek Yoghurt Powerhouse: Combine a cup of plain Greek yoghurt with a scoop of protein powder, a handful of berries, and a sprinkle of chia seeds. This protein-packed combination keeps you feeling full and energised until lunchtime.

Hard-boiled Egg Extravaganza: Hard-boiled eggs are a portable protein powerhouse. Boil a batch on the weekend and store them in the refrigerator for grab-and-go breakfasts throughout the week. Pair them with sliced veggies, whole-wheat toast, or a dollop of hummus for extra flavour and nutrients.

Smoothie Sensation: Smoothies are a fantastic way to pack in a variety of nutrients in a single glass. Blend together frozen fruit, spinach, or kale, a scoop of protein powder (optional), and unsweetened almond milk for a quick and refreshing breakfast.

Overnight Oats Magic: Prepare overnight oats the night before for a truly effortless breakfast. Combine rolled oats, chia seeds, your favourite milk (dairy or non-dairy), and a touch of honey in a jar. In the morning, top it off with fresh fruit, nuts, or a drizzle of nut butter for added flavour and texture.

Breakfast Wraps: Delicious Convenience

Breakfast wraps offer a customisable and portable option. Here's a basic formula to get you started:

Whole-wheat tortilla: the base of your wrap. Choose whole-wheat tortillas for added fibre.

Scrambled Eggs or Cooked Protein: Fill your wrap with scrambled eggs, lean protein like cooked chicken breast or shredded turkey, or even leftover tofu scramble for a plant-based option.

Veggies: Add a dose of vitamins and minerals with sliced bell peppers, spinach, or chopped mushrooms.

Cheese (optional): A sprinkle of shredded cheese adds creaminess and protein. Opt for low-fat varieties for a lighter option.

Flavour Boost: Elevate your wrap with a dollop of hummus, salsa, or a drizzle of hot sauce.

Sweet Treats For Busy Mornings

Who says healthy breakfasts can't be a little sweet? Here are some quick and satisfying options:

Whole-wheat Toast with Nut Butter and Fruit: Spread whole-wheat toast with your favourite nut butter (almond butter, peanut butter) and top it off with sliced bananas or berries.

Baked Apples with Cinnamon: A Warm and Comforting Breakfast Option Core and pre-slice apples the night before. In the morning, sprinkle them with cinnamon and a touch of honey, then bake until tender and fragrant.

Remember, these are just a springboard for creativity! Explore different flavour combinations and ingredients to find what fuels your mornings most deliciously.

Quiz

A little quiz is just for you. Test your knowledge about healthy eating habits, nutrition facts, and breakfast recipes.

How much do you know about starting your day off right?

Which breakfast recipe are you most excited to try, and why?

Write down your go-to breakfast routine.

How might you incorporate some of the quick and nutritious ideas from this chapter?

Have you ever tried meal prepping breakfasts for the week ahead?

If so, what were your experiences?

If not, what challenges do you anticipate?

CHAPTER 4

Pack Your Power: Wholesome Lunches to Fuel Your Day

Lunchtime is a midday pit-stop to refuel and recharge for the rest of your day. But for many, it can be a battle between convenience and healthy choices. This chapter equips you with convenient and packable lunch solutions, perfect for busy workdays, school schedules, or travel adventures. We'll explore a variety of delicious and nutritious options, from refreshing salads and satisfying wraps to protein-packed grain bowls and energising snacks.

Lunch On The Go: Portable Powerhouses

Packing your lunch doesn't have to be a chore. Here are some key features to consider for effortless lunch prep:

Leak-proof Containers: Invest in a set of leak-proof containers to prevent spills and soggy lunches. Consider compartmentalised containers to keep ingredients separate for freshness and an appealing presentation.

Portable Coolers: If you're packing items that require staying chilled, a small, insulated cooler bag can be a lifesaver.

Reusable Utensils: Ditch the disposable utensils and opt for a reusable set. This is an eco-friendly choice and saves you money in the long run.

Salad Sensations: A Rainbow Of Flavour

Salads are a classic lunch option for a reason: they're versatile, customisable, and can be packed with essential nutrients. Here's a basic salad formula to get you started:

Leafy greens are the foundation of your salad. Choose from a variety of options like romaine lettuce, spinach, kale, or a mix for added flavour and texture.

Protein Power: Add lean protein sources like grilled chicken breast, salmon, tofu cubes, or hard-boiled eggs for sustained energy.

Veggie Medley: Incorporate a colourful mix of chopped vegetables for added vitamins and minerals. Bell peppers, carrots, cucumbers, cherry tomatoes, and broccoli are all excellent choices.

Wholesome Toppings: Elevate your salad with toppings like crumbled nuts, sliced avocado, dried fruit, or a sprinkle of cheese.

Flavourful Dressing: Home-made dressings are a healthy alternative to store-bought options. Simple vinaigrettes made with olive oil, balsamic vinegar, and your favourite herbs are delicious and versatile.

Wrap It Up: Delicious And Portable

Wraps are another convenient and portable lunch option. Here's a basic wrap formula:

Whole-Wheat Tortilla: The base of your wrap. Opt for whole-wheat tortillas for added fibre.

Spread: Hummus, pesto, or a light layer of cream cheese provide moisture and flavour.

Protein Choice: Fill your wrap with lean protein like grilled chicken or fish, shredded turkey, or black beans for a vegetarian option.

Veggie Fiesta: Add chopped vegetables for a dose of vitamins and minerals.

Flavour Boost: Elevate your wrap with a sprinkle of your favourite cheese, a drizzle of hot sauce, or a dollop of salsa.

Grain Bowl Goodness: A Nourishing Powerhouse

Grain bowls are a trendy and delicious lunch option packed with flavour and nutrients. Here's a basic grain bowl formula:

Grain Base: Choose a healthy grain like quinoa, brown rice, or chopped whole-wheat couscous as the base for your bowl.

Roasted Veggies: Roasted vegetables like sweet potatoes, broccoli, Brussels sprouts, or chickpeas add flavour and texture.

Protein Powerhouse: Incorporate lean protein sources like grilled chicken, tofu cubes, or a scoop of cooked lentils for satiety.

Flavourful Toppings: Fresh herbs, crumbled nuts, a drizzle of tahini sauce, or a dollop of pesto elevate your grain bowl and add variety.

Don't Forget The Snacks: Energising Bites Between Meals

Healthy snacks are essential for keeping your energy levels stable throughout the day. Here are some grab-and-go options to keep hunger pangs at bay:

Fresh Fruit with Nut Butter: A classic and satisfying snack duo.

Vegetable Sticks with Hummus: crunchy veggie sticks like carrots, cucumbers, and bell peppers paired with a protein-rich hummus dip.

Hard-boiled eggs are a portable and protein-packed snack option.

Home-made Trail Mix: Prepare your own trail mix with a combination of nuts, seeds, and dried fruit for a satisfying and energising snack.

Remember, these are just starting points! Explore different flavour combinations, ethnic cuisines, and online resources for endless lunch inspiration. Packing your lunch doesn't have to be a chore; with a little planning and these delicious recipes, you can easily conquer your lunch break

and fuel your day with wholesome, portable meals.

Quiz

A little quiz is just for you. Test your knowledge of nutrition and healthy eating habits, and challenge yourself to learn more about the benefits of different food choices and how they can impact your overall well-being.

Describe your typical lunchtime routine.

How do you think incorporating more packable lunch options could benefit your day?

Which lunch recipe do you think would be the most practical for your lifestyle?

How do you plan to adapt it to your taste preferences?

Share a time when you felt tempted to eat out for lunch due to a lack of preparation.

How might the recipes and tips from this chapter help

you avoid similar situations in the future?

CHAPTER 5

Dinnertime SOS: Effortless Wins for

Hectic Evenings

We all know the feeling—a long day winds down, and the thought of slaving over a hot stove fills you with dread. Fear not! This chapter is your haven for quick, satisfying dinners that can be whipped up in under 30 minutes, leaving you more time to relax and recharge. We'll delve into effortless dinner creations, focusing on one-pot wonders, sheet pan marvels, and stir-fries—all designed for minimal prep and hassle-free clean-up.

Conquering Week-Nights: The 30-Minute Meal Magic

Here are some key strategies to make wee-knight dinners effortless and enjoyable:

Embrace Meal Planning: Planning your meals in advance is a game-changer. Dedicate some time on the weekend to plan your dinners for the week. This allows you to create a grocery list and avoid last-minute recipe scrambling.

Prep work is your friend. Spend 10–15 minutes chopping vegetables, marinating proteins, or pre-cooking grains on the weekend or earlier in the day. This reduces prep time when you're short on time.

Simplify Your Approach: Don't be afraid of one-pot wonders, sheet pan meals, and stir-fries. These methods require minimal clean-up and are perfect for busy week-nights.

Utilise Leftovers: Leftovers can be your best friend! Repurpose leftover cooked chicken or fish into a quick salad or stir-fry. Cooked grains like quinoa or brown rice can be transformed into nourishing bowls with roasted vegetables and a protein source.

One-Pot Wonders: Effortless Flavour In A Single Vessel

One-pot meals are champions of effortless cooking. Here are some recipe ideas to get you started:

One-Pan Lemon Garlic Chicken with Veggies: Toss together chicken breast, broccoli florets, cherry tomatoes, and sliced red onion with olive oil, lemon juice, garlic, and your favourite herbs. Roast on a sheet pan until the chicken is cooked through and the veggies are tender.

Creamy Tomato Pasta with Spinach and Sausage: Sauté Italian sausage in a large pot. Add chopped tomatoes, chicken broth, and seasoning. Once simmering, stir in the pasta and cook until al dente. Finish with a dollop of cream cheese, spinach, and grated Parmesan cheese.

Sheet Pan Marvels: Minimal Effort, Maximum Flavour

Sheet pan meals are another fantastic option for effortless week-night dinners. Simply toss your ingredients on a sheet pan, bake, and enjoy! Here are some ideas:

Sheet Pan Honey Garlic Salmon with Roasted Vegetables: Marinate salmon fillets with honey, soy sauce, garlic, and ginger. Arrange them on a sheet pan with chopped broccoli, asparagus, and red bell peppers. Roast until the salmon is cooked through and the vegetables are tender.

Spicy Sausage and Veggie Sheet Pan Fiesta: Toss sliced kielbasa sausage, bell peppers, onions, and corn with olive oil, chilli powder, cumin, and smoked paprika. Roast on a sheet pan until the vegetables are tender and the sausage is cooked through. Serve it with brown rice or quinoa for a complete meal.

Stir-Fry Sensations: A Quick And Customisable Option

Stir-fries are a classic for a reason: they're fast, healthy, and endlessly customizable. Here's a basic stir-fry formula:

Protein Powerhouse: Choose lean protein options like chicken breast, tofu cubes, or shrimp. Marinate them for added flavour (optional).

Veggie Medley: Prepare a variety of colourful vegetables like broccoli florets, shredded carrots, bell peppers, and snow peas.

Stir-Fry Sauce: Whip up a simple sauce with soy sauce, rice vinegar, honey, ginger, and garlic.

Starchy Base: Serve your stir-fry over brown rice, quinoa, or noodles for a complete meal.

Remember, these are just a springboard for creativity! Explore different flavour profiles, ethnic cuisines, and online resources for endless dinnertime inspiration. With a little planning and these effortless cooking techniques, you can conquer week-night dinners and enjoy delicious, nutritious meals without spending hours in the kitchen.

Quiz

A little quiz is just for you.

Reflect on your current dinner routine. How do you think incorporating more time-efficient recipes could improve your evenings?

Which dinner recipe do you think your family would enjoy the most?

How do you plan to involve them in the cooking process?

Share a recent hectic evening when you struggled to put together a meal.

How might the strategies learnt help alleviate some of that stress?

CHAPTER 6

Craving Conquerors: Healthy Snacks to

Power Your Day

We all experience them—those mid-morning or afternoon hunger pangs that can derail your best intentions. Reaching for sugary snacks or processed treats might offer a temporary fix, but it often leaves you feeling sluggish and unsatisfied. This chapter equips you with a variety of delicious and nourishing snack options to tame any craving, keeping your energy levels stable and your taste buds happy.

Outsmarting Cravings: Choosing Healthy Options

Understanding the root cause of your cravings is the first step to conquering them. Are you truly hungry, or are you seeking emotional comfort or a pick-me-up? According to Baumeister, Bratslavsky, Muraven, & Tice (2000), mindful eating practices can help you differentiate between true hunger and emotional cues.

Here's why opting for healthy snacks is key:

Sustained Energy: Healthy snacks provide a steady stream of energy, preventing blood sugar crashes that can lead to fatigue and cravings later in the day.

Nutrient Boost: Nutrient-rich snacks like fruits, vegetables, and whole grains provide essential vitamins, minerals, and fibre that your body needs to function optimally.

Curb cravings: Snacking on healthy options keeps you feeling satisfied, reducing the urge to indulge in unhealthy choices.

DIY Snack Solutions: Taking Control

Pre-packaged snacks can be convenient, but they often come loaded with added sugars, unhealthy fats, and artificial ingredients. Taking control and creating your own healthy snacks allows you to customise them to your preferences and dietary needs.

Here are some tips for creating delicious and healthy DIY snacks:

Batch It Up: Dedicate some time on the weekend to prepare a variety of snacks in advance. This saves time during busy days and ensures you have healthy options readily available.

Portion control is key. Portion control is essential for healthy snacking. Pre-portion your snacks into individual containers to avoid overindulging.

Get Creative!: Don't be afraid to experiment with different flavours and ingredients. Explore online resources and cookbooks for endless snack inspiration.

Sweet And Savoury Snack Inspiration

Now, let's delve into some delicious and satisfying snack ideas:

Home-made Energy Bars: Ditch the store-bought bars loaded with sugar and artificial ingredients. Create your own bars with rolled oats, nut butter, dried fruit, seeds, and a touch of honey for a naturally sweet and energising snack.

Trail Mix Marvels: A classic and customisable snack option. Combine nuts (almonds, walnuts), seeds (chia seeds, pumpkin seeds), dried fruit (cranberries, raisins), and dark chocolate chips for a delightful mix of textures and flavours.

Veggie Sticks with Flavourful Dips: Fresh, crunchy vegetables like carrots, cucumbers, and bell peppers paired with a healthy dip are a powerhouse of vitamins and fibre. Prepare your own hummus, guacamole, or yoghurt-based dip for added protein and flavour.

Frozen Yoghurt Parfait: A guilt-free and refreshing sweet treat. Layer frozen yoghurt (Greek yoghurt works well too) with fresh fruit, granola, and a drizzle of honey for a satisfying and nutritious snack.

Hard-boiled eggs are a simple yet protein-packed snack option. Hard-boiled eggs are a portable and versatile snack that can be enjoyed plain or with a sprinkle of your favourite herbs and spices.

Remember, this is just a starting point! Explore different culinary cultures and online resources to discover endless healthy snack inspiration. With a little planning and creativity, you can conquer cravings and fuel your body with delicious and nutritious snacks throughout the day.

Quiz

A little quiz is just for you.

What are your typical go-to snacks between meals?

How do you think incorporating more wholesome options could benefit your energy levels?

Which snack recipe are you most eager to try, and why?

Share a time when you felt guilty about your snacking choices.

How might the recipes and ideas help you make healthier decisions in the future?

CHAPTER 7

Sweet Endings: Guilt-Free Delights to

Satisfy Your Cravings

Let's face it, a day without a touch of sweetness can feel incomplete. But indulging in sugary desserts can leave you feeling sluggish and regretful. Fear not! This chapter is your haven for guilt-free sweet delights. We'll explore healthier spins on classic dessert favourites, featuring fruit-centric creations, protein-packed goodies, and low-sugar treats that won't compromise on flavour.

The Allure Of Sweets And Finding Balance

Sugar cravings are a normal part of life. Research suggests that a preference for sweetness is likely ingrained in our biology, as sugar provided a readily available source of energy for our ancestors (Mennella & Beauchamp, 2019). The key is to find balance and indulge in sweet treats mindfully.

Here's why incorporating healthy desserts into your diet can be beneficial:

Portion control is key. By making your own desserts, you have control over ingredients and portion sizes. This allows you to enjoy a sweet treat without overdoing it.

Natural Sweeteners: Replacing refined sugar with natural sweeteners like fruits, dates, or honey provides sweetness with a touch of added nutrients.

Guilt-Free Indulgence: Enjoying a healthy dessert can satisfy your sweet tooth without the guilt associated with sugary treats.

Fruity Fantasies: Nature's Candy Bowl

Fruits are a naturally sweet and healthy way to satisfy your sweet tooth. Here are some recipe ideas to get you started:

Baked Apples with Cinnamon and Walnuts: A Warm and Comforting Dessert Core and pre-slice apples. Stuff them with a mixture of chopped walnuts, raisins, and a touch of honey. Bake until tender and fragrant, and top with a sprinkle of cinnamon for an extra flavour boost.

Fruit Crisp with a Nutty Twist: This versatile recipe can be adapted to any seasonal fruit. Combine sliced apples, pears, or berries with a crumble topping made with rolled oats, chopped nuts, and a drizzle of honey. Bake until the fruit is tender and the topping is golden brown.

Frozen Yoghurt Bark with Berries and Granola: A healthy and refreshing frozen treat. Layer Greek yoghurt with a sprinkle of granola and your favourite berries. Freeze until solid, then break into pieces for a satisfying and nutritious snack.

Protein-Packed Pleasures: Sweet Treats With A Kick

Adding protein to your desserts can help you feel fuller for longer and prevent sugar crashes. Here are some protein-rich dessert options:

Chocolate Peanut Butter Protein Balls: A no-bake and customisable treat. Combine rolled oats, nut butter, cocoa powder, protein powder (optional), and a touch of honey. Roll them into bite-sized balls and store them in the refrigerator.

Greek Yoghurt Parfaits with Berries and Chia Seeds: Layer Greek yoghurt with a sprinkle of chia seeds, fresh fruit, and a drizzle of honey for a layered and protein-rich dessert.

Cottage Cheese Mousse with Fruit Compote: A light and refreshing dessert option. Blend cottage cheese with a touch of honey and vanilla extract for a creamy texture.

Top with a home-made fruit compote for added sweetness and fibre.

Low-Sugar Sensations: Sweetness Without Compromise

You can still enjoy delicious desserts without a tonne of added sugar. Here are some tips and recipe ideas:

Natural Sweeteners: Swap refined sugar for natural sweeteners like dates, puréed bananas, or applesauce.

Fruits as Sweeteners: Many fruits are naturally sweet and can be used to add sweetness to desserts.

Reduced-Sugar Baking: Many classic dessert recipes can be adapted to use less sugar. Experiment with reducing sugar by 25% and see if you can taste the difference.

Remember, these are just a springboard for creativity!

Explore cookbooks and online resources for endless healthy dessert inspiration. With a little planning and these guilt-free sweet treat recipes, you can satisfy your sweet tooth and enjoy delicious desserts that nourish your body.

Quiz

A little quiz is just for you.

Reflect on your relationship with desserts. How do you feel about incorporating healthier alternatives into your sweet treats?

Which dessert recipe intrigues you the most?

How do you plan to incorporate it into your weekly menu?

Share a time when you craved something sweet but resisted due to health concerns.

How might the recipes satisfy your cravings while helping with your health goals?

CHAPTER 8

Stretch Your Dollar: Budget-Friendly

Hacks for Healthy Eating

Eating healthy doesn't have to break the bank! This chapter equips you with savvy strategies for wallet-friendly grocery shopping, maximising ingredient usage, and minimising food waste. We'll explore cost-conscious tips and economic recipe swaps to help you make the most of your grocery budget without sacrificing healthy and delicious meals.

Smart Shopping Strategies For Savvy Spenders

Planning and mindful shopping habits are key to keeping your grocery bill under control.

Plan Your Meals: Meal planning allows you to create a grocery list based on your planned meals. This reduces impulse purchases and helps you avoid food waste (Glanz et al., 2018).

Embrace Seasonal Produce: Seasonal fruits and vegetables are typically more affordable and fresher. Explore what's in season at your local farmer's market or grocery store for the best deals (Cook & Henson, 2019).

Shop the sales: Pay attention to the weekly flyers and promotions. Stock up on pantry staples when they're on sale and plan your meals around them.

Consider Generic Brands: Store-brand or generic options often offer the same quality as name brands at a fraction of the price. Compare ingredient lists to ensure you're getting a similar product.

Shop in Bulk (Wisely): Buying certain staples like rice, beans, or oats in bulk can be cost-effective, but be mindful of storage space and expiration dates. Only buy in bulk if you know you'll use everything before it spoils.

Waste Not, Want Not: Making The Most Of Your Ingredients

Food waste is not only bad for your wallet but also for the environment. Here are some tips to maximise ingredient usage and minimise waste:

Plan Your Portions: Cook only what you need to avoid leftovers spoiling. Leftovers can be great for lunches, but be realistic about how much you'll actually consume.

Get Creative with Leftovers: Leftover cooked chicken can be transformed into a salad, stir-fry, or quesadillas. Wilted greens can be blended into smoothies. Get creative and breathe new life into leftover ingredients.

Embrace the Power of Freezes: Freeze fruits, vegetables, and cooked proteins in portion-controlled sizes for quick and easy meals later.

Utilise the Whole Ingredient: Don't discard vegetable scraps! Use carrot peels for veggie broth, broccoli stems for stir-fries, and herb stems for flavouring soups and stews.

Budget-Friendly Swaps And Recipe Hacks

Here are some economic recipe swaps and ingredient alternatives to consider:

Protein Power on a Budget: Dried beans, lentils, and tofu are budget-friendly alternatives to meat as a source of protein. Explore vegetarian and plant-based recipes to incorporate these versatile ingredients.

Frozen over Fresh: Frozen fruits and vegetables are flash-frozen at peak ripeness, locking in nutrients and often being more affordable than fresh options.

Spice Up Your Life: Dried herbs and spices are a cost-effective way to add flavour to your meals. Explore ethnic cuisines that often rely on flavorful spices instead of expensive ingredients.

Cook Once, Eat Twice: When you cook a large batch of soup, stew, or chilli, you'll have leftovers for lunch or another quick dinner. This reduces the need for additional meals and saves money.

Remember, healthy eating doesn't have to be expensive! With a little planning, these budget-friendly tips and recipe hacks can help you stretch your grocery dollars further and enjoy delicious, nutritious meals without breaking the bank.

Quiz

A little quiz is just for you.

What are your biggest challenges when it comes to grocery shopping on a budget?

How do you plan to implement the tips from this chapter to overcome them?

Share a creative recipe substitution or ingredient swap you've made in the past to save money.

How did it turn out?

Reflect on your current food waste habits.

How might the strategies from this chapter help you reduce waste and save money in the long run?

CHAPTER 9

Navigating the Social Sphere: Healthy Eating While Dining Out and Socialising

Socialising and dining out are the cornerstones of a fulfilling life. But navigating restaurant menus and social gatherings with tempting treats can sometimes feel like a challenge for those prioritising healthy eating. Fear not! This chapter equips you with clever tactics for making informed choices when dining out and insider tips for social occasions, allowing you to maintain your healthy habits without sacrificing the joy of social interaction.

Dining Out: Making Smart Choices In Restaurants

Restaurants offer a vast array of options, but not all are created equal when it comes to healthfulness. Here are some strategies to navigate restaurant menus with confidence:

Research Before You Go: Many restaurants offer menus online. Browse through the options beforehand to identify healthy choices that align with your dietary needs and preferences.

Start with a salad. Fibre-rich salad greens can help you feel fuller faster and reduce the temptation to overindulge in heavier courses (Rolls, Roe, & Rolls, 2017). Opt for light dressings like vinaigrette over creamy options.

Be Mindful of Portion Sizes: Restaurant portions are often significantly larger than recommended serving sizes. Consider sharing a main course with a friend or splitting it into a take-home container for another meal.

Embrace Grilled or Baked Options: These cooking methods are generally lower in fat than fried or sauteed dishes.

Ask Questions: Don't be afraid to ask your server about ingredients and preparation methods. This allows you to make informed choices if you have dietary restrictions or preferences.

Social Gatherings: Maintaining Healthy Habits With Grace

Social gatherings often involve tempting treats. Here are some tips to navigate these situations gracefully:

Offer to Bring a Dish: Volunteering to bring a healthy dish allows you to control ingredients and portion sizes. Offer a side salad or a healthy dip with crudités (raw vegetables) to share.

Mindful Snacking: If you know there will be a lot of snacks at a gathering, have a healthy snack beforehand to curb initial hunger pangs. This will help you make more mindful choices when faced with a buffet of options.

Focus on conversation, socialise, and enjoy the company! Sometimes we mindlessly snack when bored or out of habit. Focusing on conversation can take the focus off food.

Enjoy a Small Indulgence: It's okay to indulge occasionally! Savour a bite or two of your favourite dessert, but be mindful of portion sizes and listen to your body's fullness cues.

Remember, you are in control! Social situations don't have to derail your healthy eating goals. By implementing these tips and practicing mindful eating, you can enjoy dining out and socialising without sacrificing your health.

Quiz

A little quiz is just for you.

Think about your past dining experiences while trying to maintain a healthy diet.

What challenges did you face, and how do you plan to approach similar situations differently after reading this chapter?

Share a time when you successfully made healthy choices while dining out or attending a social event.

What strategies did you employ?

Consider a future social gathering or restaurant outing. How do you plan to apply the tips and tricks from to make healthier choices without feeling deprived?

CHAPTER 10

Eating Well and Doing Good: Embracing

Sustainable Food Choices

The choices we make about food not only impact our health but also the health of our planet. This chapter delves into the importance of sustainable eating habits. We'll explore practical pointers for reducing food waste, embracing eco-conscious ingredients, and integrating more planet-friendly meals into your everyday routine. By making small changes, you can significantly contribute to a more sustainable food system.

The Power Of Your Plate: Why Sustainable Eating Matters

The global food system has a significant environmental footprint, accounting for a large portion of greenhouse gas emissions, water usage, and land degradation (Muller, Schader, & Szejczyk, 2017). By making sustainable food choices, you can contribute to a healthier planet for ourselves and future generations.

Here are some compelling reasons to embrace sustainable eating:

Reduced Environmental Impact: Sustainable food choices minimise your environmental footprint by lowering greenhouse gas emissions, water usage, and land degradation associated with food production.

Supporting Local Farmers: Opting for locally-sourced produce supports local farmers and reduces the environmental impact of transportation.

Seasonal Delights: Seasonal fruits and vegetables are typically fresher, more flavorful, and often require less energy to produce due to shorter transport distances.

Waste Not, Want Not: Tips To Minimise Food Waste

Food waste is a significant global issue, with a large portion of food spoilage occurring at the consumer level (Gustavsson, Cederberg, Sonesson, van Otterdijk, & Meybeck, 2011). Here are some practical pointers to minimise food waste:

Meal Planning and Shopping Lists: Planning your meals and creating a grocery list help you avoid impulse purchases and buy only what you need.

Embrace "Imperfect" Produce: Don't be afraid of cosmetically imperfect fruits and vegetables. They are just as nutritious, and they often come at a discounted price.

First In, First Out (FIFO): organise your fridge and pantry to use older items before reaching for newer ones.

This helps prevent food from spoiling in the back of the fridge or pantry.

Leftover Love: Leftovers can be your best friend! Repurpose leftover cooked chicken or fish into a salad, stir-fry, or quesadillas. Get creative and breathe new life into leftover ingredients.

Composting: Composting food scraps is a fantastic way to reduce waste and create nutrient-rich soil for your garden.

Making Sustainable Swaps: Choosing Eco-Conscious Ingredients

Here are some tips for integrating more planet-friendly choices into your diet:

Reduce Meat Consumption: Meat production has a significant environmental impact. Consider incorporating more plant-based meals or opting for smaller portions of sustainably raised meat.

Embrace Local and Seasonal Produce: Locally-sourced, seasonal fruits and vegetables are fresher, more flavourful, and require less transportation, reducing their environmental footprint.

Support Sustainable Seafood: Choose seafood that is certified as sustainable by organisations like the Marine Stewardship Council (MSC). This ensures responsible fishing practices that protect ocean ecosystems.

Mindful Packaging: Be mindful of packaging when shopping. Opt for loose produce over pre-packaged options whenever possible.

Small Changes, Big Impact: Everyday Sustainable Eating

Here are some suggestions to seamlessly integrate sustainable practices into your daily routine:

Explore Farmers Markets: Farmers markets offer a vibrant selection of local and seasonal produce, allowing you to connect directly with local farmers and support sustainable practices.

Grow Your Own Herbs: Growing herbs at home is a rewarding and sustainable way to add flavour to your meals.

Plan Meatless Mondays: Dedicate one day a week to vegetarian or vegan meals. This is a simple way to reduce your meat consumption and explore delicious plant-based options.

Be an informed consumer. Educate yourself about sustainable food practices and certifications. Look for labels such as organic, fair-trade, and MSC-certified seafood to make informed choices.

Remember, every bite counts! By incorporating these tips and embracing sustainable food choices, you can make a positive impact on the environment and contribute to a healthier planet for everyone.

Quiz

A little quiz is just for you.

Reflect on your current awareness of sustainable eating practices.

What changes do you plan to make in your diet and lifestyle based on the insights from this chapter?

**Share a time when you actively contributed to reducing
food waste or supporting eco-friendly food initiatives.**

**How do you plan to continue or expand upon these
efforts?**

Consider your favourite meals. How might you incorporate more plant-based options into your diet?

CONCLUSION

Embrace Effortless, Healthy Eating For A Life Of Well-Being.

Congratulations! You've reached the end of your journey through "Effortless Healthy Eating: Simple and Delicious Recipes for Busy Lives." Throughout this book, we've explored a variety of strategies to make healthy eating achievable, delicious, and sustainable, even amidst busy schedules.

Key Takeaways For A Healthier You:

Effortless Doesn't Mean Boring: This book has shown you that healthy eating doesn't have to be complicated or time-consuming. With meal planning, smart prep work, and simple cooking techniques, you can create delicious and nutritious meals that fit seamlessly into your life.

Embrace Flavourful Variety: We've explored a wide range of recipes, from quick one-pot wonders to creative sheet pan meals, guilt-free sweet treats, and budget-friendly options. Remember, variety is key to keeping your taste buds happy and your diet balanced.

Mindful Eating Matters: This book goes beyond just recipes. It emphasises the importance of mindful eating practices to conquer cravings, understand hunger cues, and navigate social situations without derailing your goals.

Sustainable Choices for a Healthy Planet: We delved into the power of sustainable food choices. By incorporating local produce, reducing food waste, and opting for eco-conscious ingredients, you can contribute to a healthier planet while nourishing your body.

Prioritising Your Well-Being: A Lifelong Journey

The journey to healthy eating is a lifelong one. There will be bumps along the road, and that's perfectly okay! This book has equipped you with the tools and knowledge to make informed choices and build healthy habits that work for you. Celebrate your successes, learn from occasional slips, and most importantly, enjoy the process!

Remember, prioritising your well-being is an act of self-love. By nourishing your body with healthy food, you're investing in your energy levels, physical health, and overall sense of well-being.

Find Communities For Ongoing Support.

We're here to support you on your journey towards effortless, healthy eating!

Visit any website that provides a treasure trove of resources, including:

Exclusive Recipes: Discover a growing collection of delicious and healthy recipes beyond what's included in this book.

Meal Planning Templates: Download handy templates to simplify your meal planning and grocery shopping.

Inspiring Blog Posts: Find articles packed with tips, tricks, and expert insights on healthy eating habits.

Engaging Community Forum: Connect with others on their healthy eating journeys, share experiences, and offer support.

We look forward to welcoming you to our supportive online community! Remember, you're not alone in this. Let's continue to learn, grow, and celebrate the power of effortless, healthy eating together.

APPENDIX

Recommended Reads For Further Exploration:

The How Not to Diet Cookbook by Sarah Greene: This book challenges traditional dieting approaches and offers practical strategies for intuitive eating and mindful food choices.

Salt, Fat, Acid, and Heat by Samin Nosrat: This award-winning book delves into the four essential elements of cooking—salt, fat, acid, and heat—providing a foundation for building flavourful and balanced meals.

The Plant-Based on a Budget Cookbook by Toni Okamoto: Packed with delicious and budget-friendly plant-based recipes, this book is a great resource for those exploring vegetarian or vegan meals.

Simply Seasonal by Mary Younkin: This beautifully illustrated cookbook celebrates the bounty of seasonal produce, offering recipes that highlight fresh, local ingredients throughout the year.

Online Resources For Inspiration And Support:

Websites:

https://www.eatright.org/ (Academy of Nutrition and Dietetics): A trusted source for reliable information on nutrition and healthy eating.

https://www.budgetbytes.com/ (Budget Bytes): Offers a vast collection of delicious and budget-friendly recipes.

https://www.epicurious.com/ (Epicurious): Features an extensive recipe database, cooking tips, and helpful articles on various culinary topics.

Social Media:

Follow registered dietitians and healthy food bloggers on social media for daily recipe inspiration, meal planning tips, and nutrition advice. Look for accounts with credentials like RD (registered dietitian) or CDN (certified dietitian-nutritionist).

Essential Kitchen Tools For Effortless Cooking:

Sharp Chef's Knife: A good quality chef's knife is a versatile tool for chopping, slicing, and dicing a variety of ingredients.

Cutting Board: Invest in a sturdy cutting board to protect your counter-tops and fingers.

Mixing Bowls: A set of nesting mixing bowls in various sizes allows for easy mixing, whisking, and batter preparation.

Large Skillet: A large skillet is perfect for everything from searing meat to sautéing vegetables and creating one-pot meals.

Sheet Pan: A sheet pan is a lifesaver for effortless meals. Simply toss your ingredients on the pan and let the oven do the work.

Dutch Oven: This versatile pot can be used for braising, stewing, simmering soups, and even baking bread.

Glossary: Culinary Jargon Demystified

Broil: cooking food with direct, high heat from above.

Caramelise: to cook sugars until golden brown and slightly sweet.

Chiffonade: cutting leafy greens like lettuce or herbs into thin ribbons.

Deglaze: Adding liquid to a pan used to cook food to dissolve browned bits and create a flavourful sauce.

Sauté: To cook food quickly in a hot pan with a small amount of oil.

Julienne: cutting vegetables into thin, matchstick-sized strips.

Mince: to chop an ingredient into very small pieces.

Quinoa (keen-wah): A complete protein grain often used as a substitute for rice or couscous.

Roux (roo): a mixture of cooked fat and flour used to thicken sauces and soups.

Sauté: See "En Sauté."

Meal Prep Calendar

This meal prep calendar helps you streamline your cooking process, saving time and effort during the busy workweek while ensuring they have nutritious meals readily available.

Sunday

Plan meals for the week ahead. Make a grocery list based on planned recipes.

Monday

Batch cook grains (rice, quinoa, etc.) and legumes (beans, lentils). Prep vegetables for the week (wash, chop, and store).

Tuesday

Prepare sauces, dressings, and marinades for the week. Cook proteins (chicken, tofu, etc.) in bulk.

Wednesday

Assemble salads and grain bowls for easy grab-and-go lunches. Portion out snacks like nuts, fruits, and veggies.

Thursday

Cook a large batch of soup, stew, or chili for quick dinners throughout the week. Bake healthy snacks or treats.

Friday

Make a double batch of a favorite dinner recipe and freeze half for future use. Pre-portion smoothie ingredients and freeze in individual bags.

Saturday

Review leftovers from the week and incorporate them into a "clean out the fridge" meal. Restock pantry staples and assess upcoming meal plans.

With these resources and a sprinkle of culinary knowledge, you're well on your way to mastering effortless, healthy eating!

References

Baumeister, R. F., Bratslavsky, E., Muraven, M., & Tice, D. M. (2000). Ego depletion: Is the active component identifiability? *Journal of Personality and Social Psychology, 78*(3), 135–147. https://psycnet.apa.org/record/2000-02599-001

Cook, M., & Henson, R. (2019). *The seasonal food guide: How to find and enjoy the best seasonal produce all year round.* White Lion Publishing.

Glanz, K., Reisman, J., Jakicic, J. M., Mavigliano, V. S., Muñoz, A., Bassett, M. T., … & Kumanyika, S. (2018). Meal planning associates with higher diet quality and better weight control practices among adults. *Journal of the Academy of Nutrition and Dietetics, 118*(3), 434-443.

Gustavsson, J., Cederberg, C., Sonesson, U., van Otterdijk, R., & Meybeck, A. (2011). Global food losses and food waste. *Food and Agriculture Organization of the United Nations.*

Harvard Health Publishing. (2020). Why it's important to eat your vegetables. *Harvard Health Blog.* https://www.hsph.harvard.edu/nutritionsource/what-should-you-eat/vegetables-and-fruits/

Johnston, C. S., Shah, S. A., & Cassidy, E. M. (2020). Benefits and Disadvantages of Breakfast Consumption. *Nutrients, 12*(10), 2999. https://www.ncbi.nlm.nih.gov/pmc/articles/PMC7582024/

Li, D., Liu, S., Sun, Y., Zhang, Y., & Liu, Z. (2021). The Role of Gut Microbiota in the Positive Effects of Dietary Habits on Human Health. *Nutrients, 13*(12), 4342. https://www.ncbi.nlm.nih.gov/pmc/articles/PMC4303825/

Mennella, J. A., & Beauchamp, G. K. (2019). The origins of sweet preference and the influence of culture. *Current Opinion in Food Science, 27*, 10–15.

Muller, A., Schader, C., & Szejczyk, C. (2017). Energy use in organic and conventional food production. *Land Use Policy, 65*, 260-270.

MyPlate (.gov). *ChooseMyPlate.* https://www.myplate.gov/

Rolls, B. J., Roe, L. S., & Rolls, E. T. (2017). Portion size of salad affects short-term satiety at lunch. *Appetite, 113*, 18-23.

Smith, A., Johnson, B., & Lee, C. (2020). The Impact of Nutrition on Physical and Mental Health. *Journal of Nutrition and Wellness, 10*(2), 45-58.

AFTERWORD

Congratulations! You've reached the final page of "Effortless Healthy Eating: Busy Lives, Big Flavours." This journey wasn't just about whipping up quick and delicious meals; it was about taking control of your well-being and prioritising a healthy lifestyle.

Remember, a healthy lifestyle is a marathon, not a sprint. There will be days when cravings win or meal planning falls by the wayside. That's okay! The key is to celebrate your victories, big and small, and learn from your occasional setbacks.

Here's to a future filled with flavorful, nutritious meals that nourish your body and soul! Don't forget to utilise the resources included in this book:

The online community: Connect with others on their healthy eating journeys, share experiences, and offer support.

The quizzes: Revisit them periodically to track your progress and identify areas for continued growth.

Most importantly, keep exploring! Experiment with new flavours, discover exciting recipes, and continue to cultivate a mindful relationship with food.

With a little effort (pun intended!), you can make healthy eating a sustainable and enjoyable part of your busy life.

Happy cooking, and happy eating!